BEHIND T

True Stories From the Nursing Home
And How God Showed Up

by J.P. Landers

Includes a Practical Guide On How To Choose A
Nursing Home

It's Not About Them

There are wonderful doctors, nurses and therapists that are absolutely vital in the nursing home industry. In fact they are irreplaceable. The comprehensive care they provide, the long, unplanned hours they stay on shift; and the going above and beyond efforts truly save many patients. But this book isn't about them. It's about the ways in which nursing homes still need to be improved; in their process, with staffing issues and basic responsiveness to patient care. We need good nursing homes to take care of those that cannot be cared for any other way. But it will take an honest look at the situations that fail some patients before we all put the effort into transforming the nursing home industry. It can be done!

Foreword

The stench, putrid and strong, slams me in the face as the front doors swing open and I cross the threshold. That odor is what I will always remember, that distinct smell of a nursing home. Some said they got used to it but I never did. I tried but couldn't. Thus far I've managed to spend twenty years providing therapy to patients in those buildings, amidst the sour odors and other noxious encounters.

Despite misconceptions, there are some very caring and loving professionals working in nursing homes; dedicated doctors, astute professional minded nurses, and warm hearted certified nurses aides (CNA's). CNA's are an important foundation in the hierarchy of the nursing home. Rehab therapists know this and depend on them to follow through with instructions for their patients. Sadly though, in most cases, they are under trained, under paid and through no fault of their own, are mal-equipped to handle the patients they are assigned.

So often the good and positive events occurring within the nursing home become buried under layers of incompetence and negative attitudes that permeate like the plague. Unpleasant conditions prevail; sickness, debilitation, neglect and death. During my years of being licensed in rehab therapy, most people I met when discovering my career gave me a blank stare and asked, 'How do you do it?'.

That's precisely what led me to write this book. Because how I did it was not in my own strength at all. Too many hopeless conditions made it impossible to last on my own fortitude, and especially for as many years as I did. I tried doing it in my own strength the first eight years I practiced therapy. Dragging myself to work each morning inwardly kicking and screaming, facing patient neglect, depressing conditions, having no efficacy in changing things and feeling defeated by the enormous heaviness of it all...I hated my job.

Then in my ninth year of practicing, something incredible happened in me. Something intrinsically changed inside my spirit, mind and attitude as I came to understand and walk with Christ in a deeper and more intimate way. With this change came the bold realization that in my complaining and feelings of defeat at work...I had become numb to the wondrous, ever surprising ways God was working around me! He surprised me so much that I began to expect Him, to look for Him...even wait for Him to meet me in the difficult and heartbreaking situations I faced. Without fail He graciously joined me, drawing me to Himself, giving me His strength when I was depleted and had nothing left to give. He led me, gave me discernment and gave me endless creativity in my treatments for the purpose of helping those that He held dear to His heart. Those who desperately needed an advocate. Someone to stop, notice and care. To care enough to make a difference.

So these are the true accounts of those encounters. Actual events with real people whose identities and names have been changed and kept confidential for their privacy.

Some of the stories are more dramatic than others but all have the common theme of obeying the surprising nudges of God in order to intervene in patient's circumstances. Looking back it became clear that the Lord had me right where He wanted me in my career. Sometimes to be encouraged by God, sometimes to be inspired, sometimes to be ministered to by the Holy Spirit through the ones that were pushed aside and forgotten. And always to give of myself, to be the patient's advocate and do the tough things. To go out on a limb for them, putting my career in jeopardy for the sake of doing what's right.

For those of you who have decided to walk this life with Christ, and wondered as I had, if God really cares about the job you hold. Or wondered if He really uses you at the workplace or in that isolated corner of life you reside in that no one ever sees; let me respond boldly, 'Oh yes! Oh yes He does!". Expect Him! Wait for Him! And please read on.....

_ Alice _

She was utterly confused...every day. But for some unknown reason whenever I approached her wandering in the halls, she knew me. I couldn't figure it out. Her wrinkled face lit up, her eyes sparkled. By nursing home standards she was a resident with no potential and certainly no appeal. But to me, she was beautiful. Her old, trembling hand reached for me. "Oh honey, I know you. Do you live around here?"

"No, Alice, I work here. I stop to see you every day, remember?". Unintelligible babbling began. Words that made no sense at all as the insidious power of Alzheimer's stole her personality and any awareness of others around her. But still, there was something about Alice that brightened my day.

As time passed and Alice's condition worsened, understandable speech disappeared completely and she was having a harder time walking on her own. She was becoming totally dependent on the staff to get her up to escort her around the facility. Not a lot to ask but all too often, when a patient's status declined, the staff found it more convenient to leave the patient in bed. Many times for the entire day. With Alzheimer patients it's essential to provide a daily routine and to allow them to wander within the safety of a controlled environment in a locked building. Keeping them confined will only increase mental detachment and agitation.

Now, Alice was no longer able to wander the halls on her own or receive greetings from familiar faces. Her already reduced quality of life had become even more bare. More bleak. This upset me but what could I possibly do? I was a rehab therapist. Nursing staff didn't appreciate encroaching on their territory. The steady pull of wanting conditions to be better for the patients and the reality of knowing my suggestions would fall on deaf ears, created a professional tight rope I walked and lived every day.   Many days I took Alice home with me in my heart.

One night at home as I sat reading a book, my big lovable dog beside me, Alice came to mind. Then an idea emerged that I couldn't resist. Alice needed a big lovable dog. It just happened that my daughter had one to give away; one with long silky fur.   This would work just fine!

The next day in the rehab clinic I wrote Alice's name on the stuffed animal and set out to find her. Hoping someone had actually taken the time to get her up today, I searched the halls as people bustled about, but she was nowhere to be found. As I stopped by the community sitting room where families were visiting with patients, the room's large windows allowed brilliant streams of sunlight to flood in. Alice often sat peacefully in this room, but not today. The only place left to check was her room. I sighed and noted the time was 1:00 in the afternoon. *1:00 and still in bed.*

Knocking as I entered and opened the door, my eyes adjusted to the stark void of light. In the dark room, no lights, shades drawn tight, there was Alice laying in the bed confined by the metal bed rails. Her gray hair was rumpled and stuck to her neck. Her hands were dirty from several meals and many hours between washings. The scene pierced my heart. All the bleakness of her situation came crashing into my thoughts. Why doesn't someone care? It's not that hard! I wanted to scoop her up like a loving grand-daughter and make her day different...her very existence different.

"Alice?" "Alice, are you asleep?"

"It's me Alice, I came to see you."

Looking toward the sound of my voice but not at me, and appearing more detached than I'd ever seen her before, she babbled phrases I didn't understand.

"Mumble, mumble." She wasn't aware of my presence at all.

"Alice, look what I brought for you." Taking her frail hand I placed it on the stuffed animal, but Alice gave no response. So I guided her hand in petting the dog, but still nothing. Then slowly and very weakly she began to feel the dog's fur.

What happened next not only surprised me, but was nothing short of incredible given Alice's long standing vague mental alertness. And given that fact it had been months now since she'd even spoken a word. Ceasing her mindless babble she turned and looked straight at me with pointed clarity. Holding her breath, her eyes glistened with tears as she said, "You're just the sweetest girl; nobody treats me the way you do." Then reaching for my face, she gently pulled me to her and kissed my forehead.

I was overcome with emotion. I stood speechless. And in that instant, in a strange sort of way...I felt touched by God!

As I reflect on the occurrence that day, I can't really explain how I felt God's presence and touch. It's a mystery to me; and one that has caused me many times to ask if God is revealing himself through unlikely people in this harsh world? Does He show me His true nature and the essence of His love when I grasp the dirty, wrinkled hand of an unlovable person?

"Many oh Lord my God, are the wonders You have done."
Psalm 40:5

_ Clara _

Nursing homes don't always house the old and dying. At fifty-four years of age, Clara was neither old nor was she leaving this world anytime soon. Diabetes had stalked her most of her life, robbing her of sight and more recently, stealing her right leg. After the amputation surgery she needed rehabilitation. So she arrived at the nursing home a few days later. Her records arrived as well, with a dreaded label stamped on the chart...'PERMANENT ADMISSION'.

I liked Clara from the very beginning. Though uneducated she was bright, carefree and funny. We often laughed our way through therapy. Clara always put forth maximum effort, despite the inevitable fact that she was never leaving this place. Physically she was pretty amazing as we worked on her strength and mobility. Quite early in her rehab program it became clear that she was a prime candidate for returning home to live independently. But I hadn't spoken a word to her yet...it wasn't time. First I had troubled waters to navigate with that 'PERMANENT ADMISSION' issue. Day after day I pushed her harder.

One rainy day Clara seemed quiet. After the treatment I asked her about it.

"What's the matter Clara?"

"Oh, I guess I'm just missing Thomas." Thomas was her new husband of one year. An unusual marriage by any standards. She a blind amputee marrying a mentally handicapped man. As unorthodox as it was, they seemed to make a good pair as they lived fully devoted to each other. Clara expressed being in love with him faithfully.

"Has he been up to see you lately?"

"No, he can't come here...it's too far. As a matter of fact, I've been thinking about transferring to another nursing home closer to my house so he can visit me."

An alarm sounded in my head. I knew this facility she spoke of and I'd worked there for a short time as a traveling therapist. It had a nasty reputation for admitting people and keeping them for years, resisting to facilitate their return to independent living, regardless of any improvements made. Because to a nursing home, losing patients equates to losing money from medicare, medicaid and insurance. I knew Clara would smother in that place. She'd be neglected and left to herself as her strength and abilities declined further into nonexistence. I just couldn't let that happen to her. The time to approach the prospect of returning home had arrived.

"Clara, there's something I want to talk over with you." She listened intently. "You're doing so well in therapy and you've progressed so far that there's a good chance you may be able to go back to live at home. If you transfer to this other facility, you may not have therapy at all, your progress and mobility will decline and you may never leave."

I was walking a fine line in how much information to divulge about another nursing home. But if I didn't give her the truth, she may be stuck in an archaic, back country nursing home for the rest of her life. And yet, sticking my neck out for her here at this facility was a risky stance to take as well, when administration had admitted her with permanent funding to follow her arrival. Territorial egos would not appreciate any nudging from therapy on this. But I felt compelled to go to bat on her behalf and hoped that God would do what I was sorely lacking here...the ability to change things for her future. Wouldn't I want someone to do the same for me if I were in her shoes? No matter the confrontation, no matter the outcome, I had to try!

"Clara, would you like to be able to go home instead?"

"Oh, more than anything in the world! But they told me when I came here that I'd never go home again. They told me I'd be here...from now on."

"Well, keep this conversation just between us and give me some time to work on it, ok? I'll see what I can do."

That afternoon I made my way into the admitting office and faced the stern, authoritative woman that held the balance of so many patients lives in her hands. This woman that will go to her comfortable home at the end of each work day, while controlling the destiny of the patients here. Obviously irritated at my presence; and becoming more miffed as my conversation took full flight; she stood facing me with steely eyes. Barely able to wait for me to finish explaining why Clara was appropriate for returning home, she looked at me with chilly resolve.

"But she was admitted as a long term placement." Then she turned her back making the point that she was done with me; punctuated with an air of that settles that!

"But" I persisted, "She may have been dependent and unable to care for herself upon admission, but now Clara is a totally different picture. She's strong, functionally mobile, performs her own self care, has good balance and is capable of living independently."

Surprised and seething now over the fact I was still standing in front of her, she came back more pointedly.

"But she has a mentally retarded husband. She can't take care of him."

Refusing to leave Clara's fate dangling in this small, musty office, I stood firm.

"Well, if that's the only reason then send her home and send HIM to a nursing home, because SHE's capable of going home!"

With no clue as to how it would all work out, I spoke not a word of my confrontation to Clara. I secretly hoped my plea had not fallen on deaf ears but had no way of knowing the outcome. I'd done all I humanly could…it was up to the Lord now. But each day when no word came; my heart broke a little more. Clara had no idea of the struggle raging inside me.

As our therapy sessions ended each day we had established a routine of wheeling back to her room; Clara propelled her wheelchair with her now strong arms, and I placed a finger on the chair to guide it, serving as her eyes. So there we were, me guiding, her pushing, and then it happened.

Clara began to sing, "Because He lives…I can face tomorrow…because He lives…all fear is gone…because I know, I know He holds the future…and life is worth the living just because He lives!"

The song washed over me like healing balm. The supernatural peace of God in that moment was so strong as He reminded me to trust Him. I swallowed the lump in my throat and wiped my eyes. "Please keep singing Clara, it's beautiful." I didn't care that everyone on our way looked up to see who was singing; I was experiencing the presence of the Lord. And so was she.

Time has gone forward and I've since been the eyes of hundreds of other patients, but none so special as Clara. What is she doing today? Oh, probably puttering around her kitchen, listening to music and feeling the warmth of her dog sitting in her lap. And Thomas? He's there too, being a devoted husband, making her happy as only he can.

Life does not fit into a neatly wrapped package. It's messy and unpredictable. A relationship that doesn't fit into the cookie cutter mold of a young, able bodied office professional, may be perfectly normal and nurturing to the maimed and handicapped couple. It's all about perspective. And the willingness to step out of the box we all want to encase our lives in to make it more controllable. Since treating Clara, I've pushed the limits of my presence and fought on behalf of many other patients. Although each time being unsure of the outcome, I've never forgotten the most important thing...because He lives I can face tomorrow!

"Be strong and courageous. Do not be afraid or terrified because of them, for the Lord your God goes with you; He will never leave you nor forsake you. "

Deuteronomy 31:6

_ Sarah _

Sometimes as a rehab therapist, I faced such extreme cases that to say I felt inadequate was a gross understatement. These cases rocked my world! Such was the patient I call Sarah.

While new to this nursing home, I wasn't quite ready for what this particular day was about to bring. Standing at my desk, I unfolded the crumpled paper referral that looked like an afterthought. Like someone had written it, tossed it in the trash and then fished it out before placing it on my desk. The reason for the referral wasn't written down. So I asked the nurse what the patient's problem was.

"Her legs." came the stilted reply, nothing more.

So I grabbed my clip board and made my way toward her room. At her closed door I knocked and introduced myself as I walked into the room. Approaching her bed I quickly assessed the silhouette of her sheet covered form, which told me she had no legs at all. She was obviously an amputee. No problem. I'd worked with plenty of amputees over the years and was already formulating a mental framework for evaluating her. I talked with her first, asking the usual questions and taking full notice of her keen mental sharpness. No dementia here. With the intention of assessing how high up the amputations occurred, I asked her permission to examine her.

Picking up the sheet that covered her body, I eased it down to get a better look only to stand there completely shocked and astounded at what I saw! I stood there beside her, speechless...my mind racing...searching for some explanation, some reason, some decent words to explain why anyone would have let this happen to her. Sarah wasn't an amputee at all....she was deformed from years of staff neglect. Both legs were bent beyond belief like two gnarled and twisted tree branches. They curled and twisted up so far behind her that the soles of her feet pressed hard against her bottom. All of her joints at the hips, knees and ankles were frozen in place. Both legs were permanently deformed into an unrecognizable jumble.

How could any decent human being with a conscience, work with this woman day after day, month and year on end while allowing this kind of negligence? It was unethical and grossly wrong. Not only are there therapeutic interventions in place to deal with her initial problem, but after a patient is dismissed from an active therapy case load, therapists should be available in every nursing home to teach the nursing and restorative staff therapeutic techniques to maintain the patient's current status. Simply put...daily range of motion, proper body positioning and effective communication could have saved her legs from this catastrophe! Now her legs were contracted into permanent deformity. Only surgical procedures would release her joints at this point. And her contractures were so severe and long standing that she would not be considered a viable candidate for surgery. Nor was she any longer a candidate for conventional rehab therapy.

I stood there still, saying nothing and hoping the horror did not reflect on my face for her to see. Inwardly praying *Lord, what am I doing here? What in the world can I possible do for her? Please give me your wisdom.*

While I was at a complete loss...Sarah looked up at me expectantly. I wanted to tell her how ashamed I was for those that failed her. I heard myself take a breath. With soft humility I began.

"Sarah, tell me what your day is like."

"Well, I eat breakfast in bed because they can't get me up anymore. And then someone baths me."

"Then what?"

"Well, that's it."

That's it...that's it? With a lifetime of dancing, children, hugs, family, roses, love of a mate and that's it? I wanted to shout or scream to make someone take this back! To do anything to make it better. But sadly there was nothing. And I knew it.

"Sarah, what's important to you? What is it you really want?"

Without hesitation and with bright enthusiasm spreading over her face the answer came. "Oh, I want to get out of this bed. I want it more than anything. I've never seen the faces that go with the voices I hear outside my room. Or seen the window that floods light into the hallway outside my door. I'd give anything to get out of this bed."

In this situation that was a very tall order. Any attempts at getting her twisted frame into a wheelchair would be impossible.

"Tell you what, I'm going to give this some thought. I'll come back to see you first thing Monday and we'll go from there."

That weekend Sarah dominated my thinking. How could I meet her request yet keep her safe in a wheelchair? They just weren't made for bodies that didn't unfold! If I put her in a wheelchair like this, essentially a human ball, her knees would hit her chin while her feet dangled in the air at seat level. With that altered center of gravity and no way to brace herself, she would hit the floor instantly.

Then I thought of an idea, a longshot at best, but worth a try. I called a carpenter friend of mine who often crafted custom pieces of equipment for me. I told him what I wanted, complete with exact dimensions and he went to work on it. The following week he delivered the piece to me and asked if he could see this in action. I was happy to show him and we set off toward the patient's room.

Sarah was eager to try the custom piece as we started installing it in a wheelchair. It was a wooden seat board that was long from back to front. It extended out about a foot longer than a normal seat, so that her dangling feet could rest on it giving her solid footing and bracing. I covered it and the sides of the chair with thick layers of foam padding. We picked up her small, rigid body and sat her in the wheelchair. Instantly she had good trunk support and a solid base of support for her feet. She neither rolled nor toppled over. It was a total custom fit just for her twisted, unusual frame. It was a success.

Sarah was joyous and elated to be sitting up in a wheelchair for the first time in years! Immediately she asked to be taken out of her room. Slowly I began pushing her out of the stale smelling room. We emerged into the hallway and what happened next is a scene I will never forget.

At once the nursing staff stopped their busy chatter and just stared at us in silence and disbelief. When they realized it was Sarah there was an eruption of applause. Everyone swooped and surrounded Sarah's chair as they began hugging her, showering her with support.

Slowly backing out of the way, I wanted her to have this moment. She reveled in their affection. Then through the tangle of arms and faces, she turned her head to search for me. With a gleeful expression of gratitude on her face she silently mouthed the words, "Thank you."

I simply grinned and nodded my head. But truly at that moment I could have turned cartwheels.

In the next coming weeks Sarah spent a lot of time in the hallways. One particular day I came out of the clinic to head home, but decided to take the long way around the hall. As I passed the spacious sitting room area, there was Sarah perched very close to the oversized picture windows. Sprays of sunshine played on her face like beautiful prisms. She sat peacefully, gazing outside.

I felt so grateful that the Lord had chosen me to help this patient who became a prisoner in her own room. One who was forgotten by most and who fell prey to the effects of years of neglect. As I prayed for guidance in an impossible situation, God was the source of creativity and ingenuity. He gave me the creativity for executing an uncommon therapeutic approach in order to give hope to one that He loved. Ideas that allowed me to change a simple element of her circumstances dramatically altered the quality of her life. How can you put a price on that? How can you explain when God shows up in the quiet corner of your life and imparts the resources and solution you needed but never could have come up with on your own?

"You Lord, keep my lamp burning; my God turns my darkness into light."

Psalm 18:2

_ Stewart _

Magical characters are rare in this life. In the ho-hum frenzy of each day many of us become so numbed by the mundane routine. We're so busy, stressed and self involved that we miss the magical and rare characters who grace our reality for a brief time.

Stewart was one such treasure, though it's hard to say exactly why. By cosmopolitan standards he was nothing special. He was not attractive with his tiny, eighty-four year old body that was grossly bent over with a curved spine. He had small, bright blue eyes and long gray hair, tinged with yellow and combed straight back. Years of neglecting his decayed teeth caused him to be self conscious and cover his smiles. His large, misshapen hands grew knobby and stiff from years of working at a jeweler's bench while earning a living. All in all, Stewart's appearance was plain and ordinary. And yet, he possessed a wonderfully gentile spirit, was happy and a pleasure to be around.

At first very weak and unable to walk, Stewart quickly responded to therapy and soon became quite mobile. Every week his strength, balance and endurance greatly increased. Despite his bent over body, Stewart worked hard. Initially what was the vague possibility of returning to independent living and going home, was now an attainable goal. He spoke often of going home, which was a far away town where he had only a few friends but no longer any family. It gave me such a forlorn feeling when week after week he had no visitors.

One Thursday morning I headed to Stewart's room, rehearsing the therapy regime I'd planned for his workout. As I knocked and entered the room, it was acutely evident that Stewart was ill. Dealing with a history of congestive heart failure, I shouldn't have been surprised, but I was. By Friday he was much worse and on Monday a strange mental fog of confusion set in.

Standing at his bedside we talked for a while before he became suddenly tired.

"Stewart, I know you feel bad so let's forego therapy today and I'll see you on Tuesday."

Looking a little embarrassed he confessed, "You know, I don't remember what day this is." With all of his physical problems, one thing Stewart never had was confusion. He was sharp. This mental fog was very new and concerning to me.

"Today is Monday and I'll see you again tomorrow on Tuesday, ok?"

With the most piercing gaze he looked at me, "Well, I'll miss you."

Suddenly I realized just how alone this man was. No family, no friends traveling to visit, no bright greeting cards, no photos, no stories from home. Just this bare room, the cold tile floor, and him. It sent a shiver down my back as I left the room. To be that alone...

Despite the fact that I was Stewart's therapist, the professional who was responsible for his medical rehabilitation; I was also his one and only visitor day after day. Though I never spoke of it, the loneliness of that reality he lived in, was for me, very pressing and heavy some days. If I had to pin down the reasons why most people hate nursing homes and don't want to even visit their loved ones when staying in one...it's that feeling of complete loneliness. It's too overwhelming for them. And when faced with it, they catch a brief glimpse into what could be their future someday, if they too fell victim to the wrong set of circumstances.

But I couldn't avoid it...I worked in and around it every day. That hard fact, coupled with many other harsh conditions of my work, is what drove me to fight against being in this profession the first eight years. I was, as the Bible says, 'kicking against the goads'. Until finally one year, my walk with Christ took on a more personal, deeper quality. And then I was able to see the wonderful people, the gems, nestled in the midst of terrible circumstances. Situations in which the Lord regularly showed up to help those people. He spoke to my heart, giving me ideas, creativity, nudgings and sometimes life saving direction that rescued a patient from death.

I was just one therapist among many. No special thing. But the last twelve years of my career I went to work on grace every day! God went with me and I learned to recognize when He was directing me. I learned the sound of His voice inside my spirit. I learned to depend on Him for solutions to impossible situations. And...I learned to recognize, when despite all human efforts to dodge it, God was taking a dear person's life out of this world, to the place where they would be free from the disease that shackled them.

While back at work on Tuesday, I was not surprised to hear that Stewart had been sent to the local hospital. Hospital is a rather generous term denoting a big medical complex with efficiency, clean sterile rooms, and bright minded doctors and nurses. Not in this little forgotten town. This hospital was commonly called the 'Back Ward'. Just the name itself conjured up images in my mind of an old, scary psych ward of yesteryear. Unfortunately that image was one and the same with this place...a dilapidated institution with dingy windows, sparse and dirty rooms with ancient equipment. The staff were scarcely seen in the halls or stations. It just gave me the creeps!

Upon hearing Stewart had been sent to the 'Back Ward' I knew instantly what I must do and do quickly. I gathered up colored paper, pens and oh yes...the nurse's camera. I constructed a giant fold out, stand up card, complete with hearts, stars and a space for a photo. All the staff I could wrangle for a photo proved no easy task, but somehow I managed to get thirteen of us in the hall with most looking confused as to why their picture was being taken. "Just trust me, I'll explain later." Plink! The flash went off and I hastily grabbed the camera and headed out the building toward my car.

For some unexplainable reason I felt a sense of urgency. I had no idea why, I just went with it as I suspected God had some reason for prompting me. The local drug store had a primitive photo printer that surprisingly spit out a clear image of our thirteen smiling faces. Adhering the photo to the card, I glanced at my watch and saw fifteen minutes remaining on my break. I pointed my car in the direction of the 'Back Ward'. Some strange and powerful drive within me wanted Stewart to be able to know that others nearby were thinking of him and that he was not alone.

On my way into the 'Back Ward' I was overcome with the bleakness that reflected in this poverty stricken hospital. Pushing that out of my thoughts, I focused on Stewart as I entered his dingy room with dirty windows. When he saw me the surprise beamed on his face and a big grin spread. Stewart didn't even bother to cover his tooth decayed smile this time. His eyes had that far away look that I'd seen too many times in my job.

I couldn't resist teasing him. "Hey you...are you eating this ol' hospital food?"

"This stuff?" pointing to an indescribable blob, "It'll kill a person!"

We both laughed and made small talk.

Then I reached behind me and pulled out the giant card I'd been concealing. In this dreadful, dirty room, the bright colors of the card seemed to overpower the dead space around him. Hearts, stars and signatures of well wishes penned around the photo of thirteen smiling faces. I held the card out to him. "Stewart, we all miss you and want you to hurry up and come back to be with us!"

"Oh, my goodness, look at that." His knobby hands gently held the card as he admired its content.

At that moment I didn't see the wrinkled face, the yellow tinged hair or the smile around decaying teeth. All I saw was the brightest pair of blue eyes misting over with emotion as he smiled at me.

It doesn't seem like much, a card made for a forgotten old man in the depressing 'Back Ward'. But what would I give to feel the loving touch of God in my miserable forgotten life? If I had a depleted, lonely existence, what would I give to feel the embrace of a loving Heavenly Father? An embrace imparted through human arms. It doesn't seem like much...unless you are Stewart!

Stewart never made it out of the 'Back Ward'. At least not in the earthly sense. But he was set free! I knew he was a believer in Christ. And I also knew he went to his true home to be with the Father...and the biggest family reunion in existence waiting to greet him and welcome him home! When it's all said and done, few things really matter in this life outside of family, friends, and faith in Christ. I couldn't stand the thought of Stewart leaving this world alone, without being able to look into the face of someone who cared about him.

Giving him that simple pleasure at that moment seemed to be all that truly mattered. A small treasure for a magical character that God had given me the brief pleasure of knowing.

"Yet I am always with You; You hold me by my right hand. You guide me with Your counsel, and afterward You will take me into glory."

Psalm 73:23-24

_ Billy _

Billy came into my life one day quite by accident. After years of the staff neglecting Billy's steadily declining abilities, his referral for therapy was actually a mistake by the facility, that when discovered, the approval for therapy was quickly revoked. Disappointed I wasn't given the chance to explore helping him in therapy, I continued to visit with him every day. Most days he wheeled himself to the clinic and talked.

Billy was wonderful! He had a roaring sense of humor and lots of funny stories about growing up in the deep South, stories that were enhanced by his Southern accent. And the man loved to jitterbug. Long confined to a wheelchair, not a day passed without telling me of his dancing years. Dancing to the sound of the 'big bands' with any woman he could find! He'd quickly admit dancing the jitterbug all those years was the reason his legs wore out. He entertained me, making me laugh so much, that he could easily have been my therapist. My 'de-stress with laughter' therapist. In the midst of our visits we regularly talked about life, love, the perils of love, and of course all kinds of dancing. I grew to love Billy and would stop by his room frequently during the week just to talk.

Billy had a peculiar condition that caused me to contemplate him and the deepest heart of other people. He was African American, but had vitiligo; a skin condition causing huge areas of skin pigment loss. His otherwise very dark brown skin also had huge areas of bright pink skin and white skin...very white skin. Which color you saw in Billy was dependent upon the side you approached him from. From the back he looked to be a silver haired white man. From the front a silver haired black man. And from the side he had the distinct look of a silver haired albino. In full view he just looked like a man who was...well...a man of many colors! He used to joke with me about his colors and seemed thrilled when I dubbed him 'technicolored'. We'd both laugh as he went on to the next story. I just loved being around him.

One day he was especially quiet as he wheeled into the clinic to talk to me.

"What's wrong, Billy?"

"I'm jes a little blue."

"What's the matter?" putting down the pile of charting documentation that buried me.

"Well...I jes wish I could walk one more time. I know I'll never dance again but I miss standin' up and walkin'."

"I know Billy; if I could change that for you I sure would."

Feeling sorely lacking in helping to grant what would probably be the last dream he'd ever have, living in this facility; I knew he could never use a walker. The harsh fact was that he hadn't walked in years, sadly because someone in the nursing home allowed him to fall through the cracks and ceased to take good care of him. And the result was loss of strength, joint mobility, endurance, weight bearing ability...all necessary elements to walking. There was simply nothing I could do for him given the harsh fact they would never approve his funding for therapy. But I couldn't get him out of my thoughts. I began searching. Searching for something...anything outside the normal options of therapy equipment.

The search finally led me to an unusual piece of equipment I'd not seen before. It was called a 'Merri-walker'. It was a combination of a seat attached to a walker, all encased in a pvc pipe frame built like an open air box around the patient on all four sides. It was perfect for those patients who might be able to work on standing with a protective element for safety. The patient could sit all day if desired but when wanting to stand they simply stood. If wanting to walk they could. All this could happen at will, without the solicitation of help and with good assurance of safety while providing 'quick sitting' accommodation and preventing falls. The patient's standing and walking ability improved largely on it's own. That is if the patient could stand at all. I just wasn't sure Billy could. But I talked to him about the walker, told him there were no guarantees but that if he wanted to try one, we could. He agreed and I ordered it that day.

Weeks later the walker finally showed up at the nursing home. We quickly set about putting it together. Billy anxiously waited as he looked on, watching the entire process. By now many additional staff members had gathered around as well, curious to see if the man they regularly patted on the top of the head, was actually going to stand.

The time came to transfer him from the wheelchair to the new equipment. Once we sat him inside and latched the 'gate', we stood back and held our breath. Years of sitting in a wheelchair often robs a patient of not only the physical ability to stand but the will to do so. An expression of both anxiety and anticipation shown on Billy's face as he made eye contact with me . He hesitated...grabbed hold of the arm braces, then slowly began to raise himself up to a full standing position! To our surprise he was much taller than the rest of us. We all looked up to him and began clapping, cheering and whistling, as if he were a decorated officer receiving a medal! I've never seen such joy and pride on anyone's face. He was ecstatic.

I coached him in the mechanics of taking a few steps, trying to prepare him for the possibility of not meeting that goal since it had been so many years. But Billy was not to be held back. Somehow, after decades of being non-mobile, he took one step then two and then thirty steps before finally sitting, as we continued to cheer him on. He hugged my waist with an embrace that spoke volumes.

The rest is history. From that time on Billy was a man on the go. Forget the adjustment period, he walked everywhere and always stood while talking to anyone...looking them in the eye with pride. Billy had become a legend of sorts in the facility. He didn't come by the therapy clinic to visit me as much anymore. But that was okay, I knew he was making up for lost time.

One day I was rushing to a patient's room when I met Billy around the corner. We nearly ran head long into each other then burst into laughter at the near collision. I gave him a big hug.

"Billy, I've missed you."

"I've missed you too." deep Southern drawl sounding comforting. "I think about cha'. I was comin' ta tell ya somethan."

"And just what would that be, you man around town." I teased.

"Well, ya see, I jes wanted ta tell ya that I been in here a long time, see. Ain't no one ever gone outta their way fer me see. But you did. Ya got me this walka here and now I'm able to stand up and talk ta people again see. And it feels good. I jes wanted ta thank ya, from the bottom of my heart."

I couldn't utter a sound for the tightness in my throat. I simply smiled and reached up to hug Billy as he stood so very tall and very proud. He bent down, wrapping his arms around me and returned the sentiment.

It may not seem like a big event to most people. It didn't change his living situation, he still had to stay as a resident in the nursing home. But the quality of his life, his days...truly his moments in time, improved by exponential leaps and bounds! I was grateful that God had used me to intervene in his life. I felt such gratitude in knowing the remainder of his years would now be lived as a walking, standing man.

But two weeks later Billy left us...passing on to Glory. I guess the Lord wanted him home with Him, although in my surprise and sorrow at his sudden departure, I wished He hadn't gone...not yet. I wanted more time to talk with Billy, to share some laughs and to watch his joy as he walked down the hall.

Following that time, Billy was frequently in my thoughts. I missed him. I missed his jolly personality and his wonderful character. The funny man with the technicolor skin. I often thought of narrow minded people who refused to accept others different from themselves. And I wondered if a person were prejudiced, and held that prejudice simply on the basis of the color of another's skin...which part of Billy would they hate? His chocolate brown hand? His pink neck? His half white face? I mean after all... they couldn't possibly hate his beautiful, wonderful, colorful spirit!

"Delight yourself in the Lord and He will give you the desires of your heart."

Psalm 37:4

_ Gail _

Throughout the twenty years I spent as a rehab therapist, I'd often volunteer to take a student to train and mentor. One important concept I tried to always pass one was: your license is there to protect you, so you do your best to protect it. Yes, have fun at work; but be ethical, above board and always conduct yourself by the laws of your practice and the rules of the facility.

Little did I know such a time would come when I'd have to strictly practice what I taught my students.

Although this was my eleventh year practicing therapy, I'd been at a new facility only a week and was still feeling my way around, getting to know my co-workers and other staff.

It was a far away, back woods county nursing home. Not particularly a bad facility but the nursing staff was very lax in process and often flew by the seat of their pants. Methodology that works for a while, that is until something goes wrong. This particular day would prove to go very, very wrong.

I received a new referral to evaluate a patient who was a long standing resident in the nursing home. I knew of this patient. She was practically comatose. Literally, she could not move, not even a finger, she could not speak, move her head, roll over, nor could she open her eyes. She simply laid there month after month while staff bathed her and took care of her needs. She had recently been taken to the local emergency room for something. After a night there, she was delivered back to the nursing home.

When a nursing home patient gets sent out to an emergency room, the patient gets treated and delivered back by ambulance. Upon arrival, the ambulance drivers give a detailed report to the charge nurse on duty at the nursing home. This report contains everything pertaining to the patient: what was wrong, what the condition was at the time of E.R. visit, what they treated the patient with, and what the condition of the patient is upon delivery back to the care of the nursing home. This detailed report is in essence, a compliance record and a legal document. Not to mention, an updated report of the patient's current condition. It becomes the basis for care planning and therapy approach going forward.

With Gail's referral in my hand, I walked down the hall wondering if her comatose like status had improved. Why else would I have received a referral to evaluate her? I knew she'd been sent to the E.R. so I retrieved her chart from the rack with intentions of finding the ambulance report. *That should tell me everything I need to know, then I can go from there.* I never, repeat never evaluate a patient without looking at that ambulance report. Otherwise I'm proceeding blindly forward and could unknowingly do harm to the patient...it's just too risky.

Flipping through pages of the chart produced no report. Upon asking the nurse if the report was in another place I needed to look in, she stated it was in the chart. I looked again, more thoroughly. Nothing. I felt a strong nudging in my spirit to stick to the rules here.

Hmmm...well instead of an evaluation, I'll just have to do a 'hands off' assessment until I find the ambulance report. I'll document it in the patient's chart as to why.

Gail's door was open so I tapped and entered. She lay there seemingly coma like, just as before, no movement, no eye flutters at the sound of my voice, nothing. Both hands appeared to lay on her chest underneath the sheet.

I gently picked up the sheet to slide it out of the way, hoping to get a better look at her, since this was going to be a 'look only' assessment. When the sheet slid down what I saw made me gasp. Gail's right hand was swollen the size of a softball or grapefruit! It was dark purple and blue, and badly misshapen. I could tell just by looking that her M.P. joints (the first set of knuckles in the hand), were bent and completely out of joint!

What could have possibly happened to this poor woman? She can't move, can't speak, can't do anything for herself whatsoever! What in the world happened?

Where the heck is that ambulance report? I left the room and retrieved Gail's chart again. I checked one more time for the report but it wasn't there. Turning to the notes section, I began documenting :

"Received referral to evaluate patient but am unable to do so due to a missing ambulance report from recent E.R. visit. Performed a hands free, looking only assessment on patient, with the following observations: - Pt's right hand presents with severe edema, severe bruising and obvious dysarticulation of the MP's on the second, third, fourth and fifth digits. Will continue to look for the ambulance report from recent ER visit, but will NOT evaluate patient without the report."

Now, here's the thing... I knew that if and when the staff read my note, I was going to become someone's worst enemy. But if I said nothing, it would be not only cruel to Gail, but it would be completely unethical! I was sorry the report was missing...for Gail, for the staff and for myself. I wanted to be a well liked therapist on the floor. But the fact remained it was missing and that took precedence over all. And if I'd evaluated her without that report, then I would be the cause and bare the liability of her hand's horrendous condition. Someone, somewhere knew exactly what had happened to Gail. I was sorry that my documented honesty would ultimately be the implication of another person's guilt. But I had to do the right thing...protect my license and have it protect me.

The next morning first thing, I looked in Gail's chart for the ambulance report, but it was not there. Again I documented in the chart my observations and the missing report. That afternoon I checked the chart and checked with the nurse again but nothing.

The third day proved no better. I went to check on Gail before getting her chart. I was shocked to see a clear, small, plastic garbage bag filled with a large amount of ice, resting on Gail's hand. Someone had read my note and was trying to reduce some of the swelling and bruising. Not only was that against medical law to apply treatment without a doctor's order; but also the heavy ice on her fragile, disjointed fingers was going to make everything worse!

The ambulance report remained missing and I documented in the chart why I had not evaluated and began treatment on the patient. Again reiterating I would not evaluate this patient unless I saw the ambulance report first. After checking with nursing again, I headed back to the therapy clinic. At this point, I had not told any of my coworkers about this situation.

Back in the therapy clinic at my desk, my coworker sitting next to me, I could hear her talking to a family member on the phone.

"I was calling to let you know we stopped whirlpool on your mom today and...yes ma'am. Well she's been receiving whirlpool treatment for the past year and... Yes, for a bed sore... oh...well...she's better now so we stopped the treatment and when we do that it's customary to call the family and let them know. Ok, thank you."

"What was that all about?"

"That was my patient's daughter. We just finished a year's worth of whirlpool on her mom's ulcers and she didn't even know her mom was getting whirlpool!"

"No one called her a year ago to inform her of her mom's condition?"

"Nope. I wasn't working here then so I don't know what happened."

"Wow. Who's the patient?"

"Gail."

No...say it isn't so...this can't be happening. This situation with Gail is quickly escalating to an ugly crescendo of multiple offenses!

"Her daughter lives about three hours from here. She said she would travel to visit her mom in a few days."

Only Gail's daughter didn't come a few days later...she showed up bright and early the very next morning. I came in at seven a.m. with intentions of following up on the report situation. But as I got a glimpse of Gail's room down the hall, I saw a figure outside her door. It was Gail's daughter...standing outside Gail's closed door...while her very own lawyer inside the room was taking legal photographs of Gail!

So not only did Gail's daughter get the revelation yesterday about her mom having a bed sore for the past year; and that her mom had been receiving whirl pool for the past year... now she's getting another revelation. She showed up this morning to investigate the bed sores and got a terrible shock when she walked into Gail's room and saw the hand!

I abandoned my plan to search for the report. The dominoes would be falling into place soon enough.

After lunch while headed to the therapy clinic, I rounded the corner of the hall but was suddenly unable to pass through. From the head nurses office, down the hallway, about twenty five staff members were lined up in single file. Nurses, nurses aides, office staff. Everyone looked somber, no chatter, just silence.

Leaning in close I asked one of them, "What going on?"

"We all have to take a polygraph test!"

All day the investigation ensued, but I was never pulled into it because of my thorough documentation and adherence to the rules, despite that fact that the patient really needed immediate care five days ago. What seemed to be a random nudging from God, out of nowhere, proved to be the very thing that kept me from this scathing situation. And the Lord saw what happened to Gail. Although at the time while being totally unaware, I have to believe He used me to be a catalyst in resolving the poor treatment and negligence to which she fell victim. I thanked Him for helping Gail and me as well. It gave me hope and courage to know if I were in Gail's place, God would send someone to help me...to be my voice, to be my advocate.

"And my God will meet all your needs according to His riches in glory by Christ Jesus."

Phillipians 4:19

_ Betty _

At some point in a person's life, they may be placed in a very difficult situation. One where all that you believe to be true and good about people, comes crashing down. It is at that point you are called to step forward and do what is right, even though it may jeopardize your employment. Even though it stands a very good chance of ruining someone else's reputation and livelihood. I was placed in that position at one point in my career.

I'd only begun to work with Betty. She was new to my therapy case load but had lived at the nursing home for several years already. She had minimal capabilities of learning new therapy techniques due to having prominent Alzheimer's. Although leaving her mentally devoid of understanding, the disease had not yet developed into latter stages. Therefore my hope was to tap into Betty's automatic responses so as to illicit improving strength and mobility. After reviewing my therapy strategy for her to begin with, I started down the hall toward her room.

With my clipboard in hand and looking at my notes, I entered the room and looked up, ready to greet Betty. But someone else was already with her. And at that moment in time I wished I had not been dropped into the scene that lay before me...but I was.

Betty was dressed in merely a shirt and diaper while laying on her back in the bed, in an oblivious state as usual from the dementia. A young, male nurses aid was sitting at her feet, and while cajoling her with soft giggling, had his hand in a very private place.

It so shocked me that I stopped dead in my tracks, my mouth open as I took in the bizarre scene. What in reality was only a second, seemed like minutes as I processed what to do here. I didn't want to frighten Betty and it certainly was not my job to confront a nurses aid with accusatory statements. *Lord, help me, please show me what to do.*

The nurses aid went pale in the face as he slowly lowered his hand. His gaze was fixed on me.

I cleared my throat, " I was just going to start therapy with Betty, but I can come back." At that I turned around and left the room.

I didn't just see what I thought I saw....did I? I couldn't believe it. My mind was racing. It looked like molestation was in progress and I interrupted it! But what if it were not molestation...what if it were something else? That is a very serious charge to lay out there. A life altering charge. I walked the halls without a purpose for the next five minutes as I processed the incident and the ugly scene that I'd been instantly forced into. There was no other option...I had to tell someone. I had to, for the sake of Betty and other confused patients that lived in the facility.

As I searched for the appropriate person to talk to, my mind still reeling from the sight, I didn't quite know how to approach this. Knowing that therapists were frowned upon when sticking their nose into nursing business, I was treading on thin ice here. *God give me wisdom.*

I found the director of nursing and asked her if we could step into a private office.

"So, let me ask you a question. How are the nurses aids trained to check for soiled diapers? Diapers on female patients?"

"Well, they're trained very thoroughly," seeming defensive already. "We train them upon hiring and provide ongoing training throughout their employment."

"Mm-hmm."

"The nurses aids are trained to check for soiled diapers from the waist band and at the back."

"The back of the diaper?"

"Yes, the back." looking at me questionably, as to why a rehab therapist would be bothering her with this bit of diaper trivia. Obviously a nursing department topic and not mine to be concerned with.

"Why, what's wrong?"

"Well" I started, "I'm not accusing anyone of anything, I simply need to tell you what I saw and let you handle it from there."

The director was all ears now.

"I was going into Betty's room when........." I recounted the whole story, careful not to omit any details, also careful not to infer any details or my opinion. As a witness to the scene, I needed to relay details and let her take the situation into her own hands to deal with properly.

The Director's face turned red, her lips pressed tightly together. "Ok, thank you very much for telling me."

That was it. The Director never got back to me, never followed up to tell me anything else. Because nurses aids were accountable to and supervised by the nursing department. But, that particular young, male nurses aid was not there the next day or any other day following. I could only surmise he was let go after an inquisition revealed his misconduct.

It is common and rightly so, to think that residents in nursing homes are helpless and unable to defend themselves. They have to depend on others to do for them; to do simple tasks that we healthy people take for granted. Employees that the patients must depend on, can run the entire spectrum of moral character, from good and caring to mean and cruel. But through years of providing therapy to nursing home patients, I learned that even the most helpless patient is never alone. They always have a loving, empathetic heavenly Father who cares about them. He witnesses all... oversees their plight, and sometimes sends in an earthly advocate to step in and be their voice. Though harsh and shocking as this incident was, God used it not only to come to Betty's aid, but also to bolster the faith of a young therapist. He strengthened my faith in Him to know He would always be there for others including me, working out solutions on our behalf...even when it seems impossible.

"I have told you these things, so that in Me you may have peace. In this world you will have trouble. But take heart! I have overcome the world."
John 16:33

_ Clark _

He pushed his own wheelchair into the clinic, presenting himself ready for the day's therapy. Unlike the others in rehab that day, Clark was making great progress toward going home soon.

You couldn't know Clark without falling in love with his infectious smile, twinkling eyes and his warm accepting manner. A big man, burly and muscular; he commanded attention just sitting in the room. He was the gentle giant...a rock of a man, yet always ready to help someone else. In the clinic when rehab therapy demanded more than a patient felt they could give, Clark wheeled over to them at the machine with words of encouragement.

"Now you can do this! When I was at the place you are now and I thought I couldn't go on anymore, I just kept pushing myself. Then I got better. Come on now, you can do it!"

He was a naturally gifted leader...even in the nursing home. Other patients responded to him, followed him. When a patient was too ill to get out of bed, Clark wheeled into the patient's room, prepared to give them a bedside chat. He had all the great bedside manner of a good doctor and then some!

Clark fit right in with our rehab team. This unusual team of therapists; colleagues I had been so blessed to work with, were very atypical. Not the common mix of pessimists and downers, causing drama for everyone...far from it! They were fun to work with, conscientious about delivering good therapy, supportive of the others and most unusual...they were down right hilarious! No matter the day, no matter the difficulty, we all had such a good time talking, joking and always laughing. Even the patients would say, "This is the only place where it feels normal, can I just hang out with you guys?"

Clark was no exception. Long after his therapy concluded for the day, you could find him in the clinic while engaged in some conversation or telling jokes. Many times bringing other patients with him that needed a friend. We grew accustomed to Clark's own way of social networking.

Although his progress in rehab was nearing a close with the prospect of returning home in his sights...there was something that left me feeling unsettled...a foreboding feeling. You see Clark had a very large abdomen. The facility doctor didn't have much to say about it when asked. Clark's outside doctor didn't have much to say about it. But even though I'm no physician, and don't pretend to have a doctor's knowledge, I'd treated thousands of patients with many conditions. And I just had a sense something was wrong.

The day before discharge came with a constant flow of hugs and lots of well wishes. Clark was beaming even more than normal. As my work day ended I stopped by his room, knowing there would be no time for goodbyes tomorrow.

"Clark, it has been such a pleasure to work with you. I'll miss you buddy".

"Oh, I'll miss you too but you'll see me again. Just as soon as I can make it back up here, I'll come to see you and the others. It won't be long."

"Well, I'm going to hold you to that. I'll look forward to seeing how well you're getting along."

Saying goodbye with a hug, I turned to leave. That unexplained, foreboding feeling still there.

The following morning as I perused my busy schedule of patients for the long day ahead, the word came. Clark wasn't going home today. He'd experienced some difficulties in the middle of the night and was sent out to the local hospital for treatment.

A sinking feeling hit me. *"Oh man...I wonder what they'll find."*

It's amazing how word spreads in a community, informally from hospital to nursing home and back, updating a patient's condition and whereabouts. Although days and weeks passed since Clark's leaving in the night, no word came of his condition or whether he was still in the hospital. Until a few weeks later.

When I inquired, the report came that Clark was coming back to the nursing home today. The hospital was performing a few diagnostic tests which would take ten days or more to get the results. So they sent him back to us for continued rehab. I looked forward to seeing him and wondered about the doctor's diagnosis.

I spotted him quite by accident sitting in the hallway, with a very obvious change from before...his abdomen had become even more distended...looking huge and deformed.

That wasn't the only change; Clark returned with an entirely different demeanor. Gone was the big burly man who presented himself in the clinic ready for comedic interaction. Someone else had wheeled Clark into the clinic. He sat off to the side of the room just inside the hallway. He made no effort to join the group but seemed content to sit alone. No jokes, no laughter, no reaching out to the rehab team or even other patients.

"Hey Clark, it's so good to see you!"

"It's good to see you too", gasping for an unencumbered breath as the large abdomen pressed on his chest.

"What's new, Buddy, and how are you feeling?"

"I'm not feeling too great. The doctor didn't have much to tell me. They ran some kind of test but I won't know the results for awhile."

We talked briefly, as I took note of the difference in Clark. In the week to follow he stayed in his bed and refused therapy, saying he just didn't feel good. Each day I passed his room, my heart went out to him and the man he used to be, knowing he was probably grieving the absence of that same man as well. And each day I passed his room, his abdomen grew bigger. Although no official word had come yet, I felt sure Clark was dealing with some kind of cancer.

A few days later as I was rushing around, treating a heavy case load of patients, I came through the opening of the clinic and spotted Clark off to the side of the room alone. He was such a big man that even as he sat in a wheelchair his head was level with my shoulders. I forced myself to stop while therapeutic plans for my next patient ran zipping through my head. On the other side of the room my colleagues were in the middle of a very funny story peppered with loud animation.

"Hey. Good to see you out of your room. How are you feeling today?"

Clark looked up, searching my eyes as though sizing me up in character somehow. The moment gave me pause. After a long hesitation he began to speak to me softly. Softly, as though touched by something serious that the rest of us were too busy to see, to hear...too busy to touch. I leaned in to hear him speak.

"You know all my life I've been the one to encourage others. I've been the one to help everyone else. No matter what the problem, if I couldn't help them with the circumstances, I could lift them up and make them feel better. I've gone into the room of lots of people and talked to them about not giving up. And sometimes I had to give them a hard talk, you know what I mean."

"I know you have Clark, you've been wonderful for so many patients here. But maybe this is the time when you focus on getting better, when you're in need of a little help now." I waited in silence knowing he had more to get out.

"But see....see... now I can't do it anymore". Emotion starting to well up. "I want to be helping them but I just can't do it... I just can't do it anymore. And if I can't do that...then what's the use in going on living like this?"

Loud, roaring laughter came from behind me, and I was struck by the irony of the scene. On one side of the rehab clinic was the epitome of a good time at work with reams of jokes, witty responses and clever one liners; followed by hilarious laughter. Juxtaposed by the other side, the side where I stood with Clark, in a deeply emotional moment, a crucial moment. A pivotal moment in time when a man assesses his worth in the reflection of life's purpose. A moment that reinforced my inadequacy, as I didn't know how to respond.

Lord, what on earth can I say to him? I'm at a complete loss here...He needs a touch from you Lord, please help me.

I kneeled down on the hard tile floor. My hand slid around his broad shoulders.

"Clark, there's a lot of things I could say to you right now. Some of them could blow off what you're feeling, some could make light of it, and some could be untrue. But the truth is...there comes a time in life when none of this other stuff...the other people in here, making them feel better...the laughter in here, the jokes...none of it really matters. The truth is that nothing else matters except your relationship to Jesus Christ...just you and Him. That's what matters now."

What happened next was truly remarkable. This big, strong hulk of a man laid his head over on my shoulder and rested there as I held him...the tears slipping down both our cheeks.

The following day he received test results showing he was positive for pancreatic and liver cancer. But Clark seemed serenely at peace.

That afternoon as he slept, one of the CNA's told me she heard him laughing in his sleep. But I knew he wasn't just sleeping... he was having a divine appointment with the living God who was giving Clark a glimpse of heaven. Clark passed on, into the waiting arms of Christ four hours later.

Jesus asked, "But what about you? Who do you say that I am?" Peter answered, "You are the Messiah."

Mark 8:29

Audry

Timid, apologetic patients sometimes fall between the cracks as they're unable to navigate through the often rough and difficult environment of nursing homes. Beyond the well furnished, polished front lobby, lies all that is good and all that is dysfunctional in nursing home processes. Wandering, confused patients invading another patient's room and sometimes their bed; noxious odors that indicate a patient has laid in soiled bed sheets far too long. And sometimes being on the receiving end of calloused, irritable help. It tests even the strong willed.

After greeting Audry and introducing myself, I took note of her keen awareness and sound mind. I explained I was going to get her out of bed to take her to therapy. With her thin little arms folded across her chest and her hands underneath her chin, she responded, "OK."

As the blanket was slid back her frail, thin body became visible under clothing far too baggy to wear. She was emaciated. Concentration camp photos flashed in my mind. Discovering she was unable to move much, I slid my arm underneath her upper back and began gently sliding her legs to the edge of the bed.

"I'm sorry" came the words as she apologetically looked into my eyes. Those two words from this frail, sweet woman made me wonder what kind of treatment she'd received.

"Sorry? What for?" I smiled at her. "Girlfriend, we ALL need a little help sometimes, it's okay."

She weighed only 83 pounds. Even though taller than me, I could literally pick her up and place her in the wheelchair. The wheelchair was juvenile sized. Still, there was lots of room around Audry's body once in the seat. According to the chart information, there seemed no real reason for her weight loss. General deconditioning and a debilitating sequence of events set about the landslide.

She also had what is called 'athetoid' movements; snake like movements in her arms and torso. They were absent when she lay in the bed. And when participating in therapy the movements only appeared to be mild. But when she became emotionally upset, the movements became prominent, large, sweeping out of control movements. In these moments, she could do nothing else with her body as the athetoid pattern dominated her other abilities.

For the next two days Audry was motivated to try in therapy, but she was so weak. On the third day as I entered her room, I could see her face was contorted.

"Audry, what's wrong?"

She could hardly speak from crying so hard. "I...I...I've lost weight again. I've been trying to eat as much as I can but the girl weighed me this morning and she said I've lost weight again," blubbering now as her arms snaked out of control.

Lord, she's only 83 pounds as it is...did she come here just to waste away till she dies? No! I couldn't believe it. I had hopes that she could improve and progress. But what could I do?

"Tell you what, try to pull it together so I can get you out of this bed, and then I'll take you myself and weigh you. OK?"

She agreed though never stopped crying. Which made the task of getting her into the wheelchair quite a bit harder as her torso and arms reacted to her state of mind.

You wouldn't think so, but the issue of weighing patients in the nursing home is a tricky one. Patients are weighed every week on a large wheelchair ramp scale. The problem is the wheelchair they are weighed in. From week to week it needs to be the same chair. Patient's assigned chairs are often swiped by other confused patients or sometimes by staff that are unwilling to walk a short distance for a wheelchair. Instead they just take the closest one. Resulting in the wheelchair that was custom fitted for a patient to turn up missing. Then in turn, any wheelchair left around is the one selected to weigh the patient in. If a patient's original wheelchair was custom fitted by therapy with certain leg rests, arm rests, a special seat cushion and an oxygen tank; it changed the overall weight of that chair. By a great deal. When some random chair falls substitute for going on the scale then the patient's weight is also off. It happens every day. And the weight gets recorded in the chart.

For many patients, weight is not such a big deal. But for Audry at 83 pounds, it was a very big deal!

I pushed her to the scale with her still crying. Instead of pushing her onto the scale and taking the reading I first transferred her out of the chair into another. Then I weighed the empty chair. I made note of the number, put Audry back in the chair and weighed her again. I subtracted the difference and discovered that Audry had not lost weight at all...in fact she had gained 2.5 pounds since the last reading. There was a possibility that last week's weight was wrong too but I had no way of knowing. So I just went with it...this lady desperately needed some encouragement.

"Audry, you haven't lost weight at all. In fact you've gained weight, 2.5 pounds. "See...it's all going to be OK!"

She began to cry more but from happiness this time. She hugged my waist as I stood beside her. Then I wheeled her to therapy and made her a hot cup of tea to sip, hoping she'd calm down.

During that time I had an idea. Surely those in charge of her care had already covered this idea but I needed to inquire about it anyway. I headed down the hall to find the charge nurse or medication nurse.

"So, I have a question about Audry."

"What's that?" not making eye contact with me but immersed in paperwork.

"Can you tell me if she is on an appetite stimulant?"

A heavy sigh proceeded as the nurse stopped what she was doing and began searching Audry's records. After several minutes she finally looked up. "Hmm, you know she's not! I have the medication list right here and I've gone over it several times. She is not on an appetite stimulant."

Medications were definitely out of my scope of responsibilities and practice. I couldn't ask the doctor to give her a medication, only the nurse could. And I get it, she was busy and didn't need my interruption pointing out what someone else had forgotten. But I also knew that Audry could possibly die without help for her failing appetite and landslide weight loss.

"Do you think you could possibly talk to the doctor and if it's not contraindicated, ask for an appetite stimulant for Audry?"

Holding my breath she responded, "Yes, I absolutely will. I'll talk to him today."

The next few weeks showed a marked improvement in Audry's condition. Her energy returned, making it possible to participate in therapy, her strength improved and her mobility improved. The best part was that she had gained 17 pounds so far and still gaining. She was well on her way to recovery and full rehabilitation! In the weeks that followed, her family made preparations for her to return home. It was going to be a joyous reunion.

The world of therapy is filled with so many stresses, that it sometimes boggles the mind. Regulations, compliance, documentation, problem solving, causing pain in patients, dealing with families in crisis and working with sometimes difficult personalities. All of this framed by rigid company expectations. But in the middle of all that craziness, God whispered in my spirit, a quiet thought about Audry. She needed an appetite stimulant to boost her caloric intake or she could slip into the point of no return. I don't know why the hospital or the nursing home didn't start her on it. Perhaps it was just an oversight. But this simple thing caused her to turn the corner in recovery; carrying a huge, positive impact for her health, well being and her very life!

It gave me such joy the day Audry was to leave the facility. She had fought against all odds, done all the hard work and climbed the mountain of impossibility! And now she was ready to receive her reward.

She came into the therapy clinic with a broad smile and proudly handed me a poem she'd written for me. While hugging me she said, "Thank you for everything you've done for me, I will never forget you." "No Audry... I shall never forget you! Thank you for giving me the privilege of working with you."

"Let the morning bring me word of Your unfailing love, for I have put my trust in You. Show me the way I should go, for to You I lift up my soul."

Psalm 143:8

HELPFUL GUIDE WHEN CHOOSING A NURSING HOME

Now, as opposed to when I first began my career, there are numerous excellent resources to tap into when searching for the right nursing home to place your loved one in. I will list some of my favorites, along with some red flags to look for and inquire about, based on my years of experience. Asking these questions, when you're under the duress of placing your family member in a facility, can be extremely helpful. These questions will slice through the nursing home's polished face presented to the public. You will be able to get right to the heart of what makes a nursing home good or bad, to make a better informed decision.

-When Visiting a Prospective Nursing Home, Ask These Questions:

- What is the ratio of CNA's to patients?
CNA is the nurses aid; they are the ones that care for your loved one hour by hour. The fewer the number of CNA's on each wing, means that patient call lights don't get answered in a timely manner, bathroom needs aren't getting the attention deserved and sometimes emergency calls don't get answered with any urgency at all. Ask for the ratio of CNA's to patients on both the day and night shift. Nursing Homes are required to post the number of staff it has at the facility, including CNA's. Keep in mind that when a facility has only one nurses aid on the wing, who's rushing from room to room, there's a good chance the facility is short staffed. This is a definite red flag. CNA's have a very important and very difficult job. They need greater support and training from the company they're employed by. They are the backbone and the beginning of good nursing care. They are the first to see your loved one in the morning and the last at night. When something is amiss with the patient, a good nurses

aid who is attentive and on the ball can alert the nurse right away. If there aren't enough aids to go around the consequences can be disastrous

- How are the CNA's trained to perform patient transfers?
Transfers refers to the manner in which a patient is moved from bed to wheelchair, from wheelchair to toilet and so on. There are safe, controlled, therapeutic techniques and equipment used to transfer patients. They should be taught to every employee and provided with the equipment needed. All too frequently a patient is accidentally dropped during a poorly executed transfer. Ask if the CNA's use Gait Belts and ask to see a demonstration. If your loved one is extremely heavy, special equipment may be needed to transfer them. Ask if the facility has a Hoyer Lift available and are the CNA's trained in using it safely.

- What is your plan for my loved one concerning urinary continence and successful bathroom use?
Patients that arrive at the nursing home with an indwelling catheter had received it during the hospital stay prior to discharge. Oftentimes the patient's initial problem is resolved and the patient can immediately be weaned from the catheter. Or the patient can enter into a weaning plan of care for catheter removal as a goal. Sometimes the catheter is not able to be removed for medical necessity. Know what that reason is and ask for explanations. Also, if the patient has a decubitis ulcer, commonly called a bed sore or pressure sore on the buttocks area, it may not heal properly while coming in contact with urine. Thus a catheter is necessary for healing. Again, know the reasons for your loved one's catheter and ask for a definite plan and steps for removing it. Catheters that are left in too long or for no reason can greatly interfere with the patient's rehabilitation.

- Why does my loved one have a pressure sore and how will you treat it?
If your loved one arrives from the hospital with a pressure sore, or worse yet develops one in the nursing home, ask for an explanation as to why.

Then ask for the plan of treatment you can expect to be administered for the healing process.

- Can my loved one be seen by therapy to provide proper positioning and seating to remove any pressure off the sore while in bed and in the wheelchair?
A good therapist can evaluate the patient and provide therapeutic intervention through positioning devices, for removing pressure to the sore while the patient is both in bed and in the wheelchair. The patient's progress can continue with this in place as it will allow the patient to participate in rehab. You can request an experienced therapist in this area, from the rehab director.

-What is your 'out of bed policy'? Will someone get my loved one out of bed every morning?
One of the patient's biggest complaints and source of frustration is being left in the bed too long with no one to help them get up and going. This wreaks havoc on the patient's well being in so many areas: they are at a high risk for developing a pressure sore which has debilitating effects; their strength diminishes, endurance wanes, balance becomes dulled, frustration sets in and their overall potential for rehabilitation is dramatically lowered. The simple act of getting a patient out of bed, in the wheelchair and into rehab therapy, can be the key to returning to independent living.

- What is your grievance policy for residents? Are they able to bring up concerns without fear of retribution?
At times patients have very legitimate concerns, when listened to by administration could be handled with an easy fix. However, if the patient fears receiving bad treatment after complaining, by the nurses aids on day or night shift, they will most likely keep silent as the problem grows and

festers. Ensure your loved one is supported by the facility in every manner.

- How is medication delivered on time when the medication nurse is behind schedule?

If your loved one has had a recent surgery, pain meds administered in a timely manner can be crucial. Therapy should communicate with the meds nurse and the patient to pick the most optimal time to engage the patient in rehab, after their pain is managed. Otherwise the patient is simply in too much pain to do anything and therapy is delayed or cancelled, just because the meds were late.

- Does this facility have a social worker or ombudsman on staff?

If a nursing home has less than 120 beds, it is not required by state regulations to have an in-house social worker or ombudsman. Usually however, the facility has an appointed employee that fills that role. They can be your best advocate when there is a serious problem. Communicate with them regularly. But in the event of a serious problem that has not been resolved by the facility first, then find out the ombudsman for your state. An ombudsman is a neutral figure who will act as a mediator between the parties that be, while acting on behalf of the patient.

Additional Resources to Look At:

- Compare the Nursing Home Deficiencies to State and National Ratings - www.memberofthefamily.net

The website has a very good checklist of all nursing homes by state and what their deficiencies are. You can compare their ratings and also view their violations in detail.

- Ask to see the Nursing Home's Inspection Report by the State -
Every nursing home has a copy of the annual state inspection report complete with violations and details. It is a public record for viewing and often is placed in the front lobby of the facility for visitors to see. If they won't provide it upon request, that is a definite red flag. If you find it too uncomfortable to request it, simply go to www.medicare.gov/nursinghomecompare   Type in the city, state and name of the nursing home you want and then click on the tabs at the top of the page, especially the tabs labeled *Staffing, Quality Measures* and *Penalties*

- Check the Medicare Guide to Select a Nursing Home -
www.medicare.gov and type in the search box:
    guide to choosing a nursing home

Made in the
USA
Monee, IL